CHEMOTHERAPY COOKBOOK

FOR NEWLY DIAGNOSED

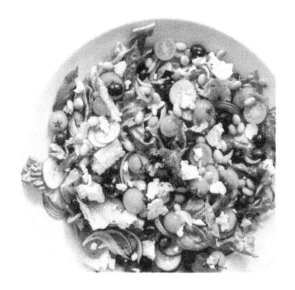

Lesa Allen

Copyright © 2024 by Lesa Allen

DISCLAIMER

This cookbook is intended to provide general information and recipes.

The recipes provided in this cookbook are not intended to replace or be a substitute for medical advice from a physician.

The reader should consult a healthcare professional for any specific medical advice, diagnosis or treatment.

Any specific dietary advice provided in this cookbook is not intended to replace or be a substitute for medical advice from a physician.

The author is not responsible or liable for any adverse effects experienced by readers of this cookbook as a result of following the recipes or dietary advice provided.

The author makes no representations or warranties of any kind (express or implied) as to the accuracy, completeness, reliability or suitability of the recipes provided in this cookbook.

The author disclaims any and all liability for any damages arising out of the use or misuse of the recipes provided in this cookbook. The reader must also take care to ensure that the recipes provided in this cookbook are prepared and cooked safely.

The recipes provided in this cookbook are for informational purposes only and should not be used as a substitute for professional medical advice, diagnosis or treatment.

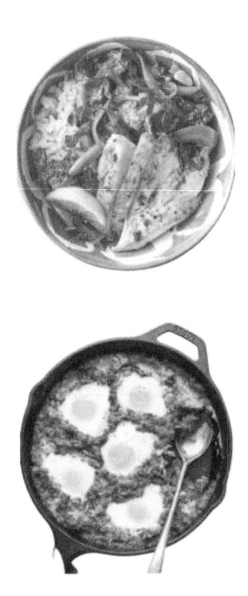

TABLE OF CONTENTS

INTRODUCTION

A chemotherapy diet is crucial for newly diagnosed cancer patients, it helps manage side effects and supports your overall health during treatment.

Chemotherapy can cause a range of side effects, including nausea, vomiting, taste changes, mouth sores, and appetite loss, making proper nutrition both challenging and essential.

Firstly, staying hydrated is vital. Chemotherapy can lead to dehydration, so you should aim to drink plenty of fluids, such as water, herbal teas, and broths.

In addition to hydration, managing nausea and vomiting is critical. Small, frequent meals that are bland and easy to digest, such as crackers, toast, and bananas, can help. Ginger and peppermint are also known to soothe the stomach.

Protein intake is essential to maintain muscle mass and repair tissues. Lean proteins like chicken, fish, eggs, and plant-based proteins such as beans and lentils should be included.

Dairy products like yogurt can provide both protein and probiotics, which support gut health.

Fruits and vegetables are important for their vitamins, minerals, and antioxidants, which can help strengthen the immune system.

However, raw produce may sometimes be hard to tolerate; therefore, cooked or pureed options might be more suitable.

Incorporating whole grains such as oatmeal, brown rice, and whole wheat bread provides necessary fiber, which helps combat constipation, a common side effect of chemotherapy.

You should also be mindful of food safety, as your immune system may be compromised. Foods should be thoroughly cooked, and raw or undercooked items like sushi or unpasteurized products should be avoided.

More so, this book is created to help you maintain strength, improve treatment tolerance, and enhance your general well-being during chemotherapy.

CHAPTER 1

WHAT IS CHEMOTHERAPY?

Chemotherapy is a cancer treatment that uses drugs as remedy to eliminate cancer cells. These drugs work by targeting rapidly dividing cells, which is a characteristic of cancer. Chemotherapy can be administered in various forms, including oral tablets, injections, intravenous infusions, or topical applications, depending on the type of cancer and the specific drugs used.

The main goals of chemotherapy are to:

1. **Cure the Cancer:** In some cases, chemotherapy can eliminate cancer completely.

2. **Control the Cancer:** When a cure isn't possible, chemotherapy can shrink tumors and stop the spread of cancer to extend life and improve quality of life.

3. **Ease Symptoms:** Chemotherapy can also be used palliatively to reduce the symptoms caused by cancer, such as pain or pressure from tumors.

Chemotherapy is often used in combination with other treatments, such as surgery, radiation therapy, or targeted therapy, to increase its effectiveness.

The drugs used in chemotherapy can affect not only cancer cells but also other rapidly dividing healthy cells, such as those in the bone marrow, digestive tract, and hair follicles. This can lead to side effects like fatigue, nausea, hair loss, and increased risk of infections.

The specific regimen of chemotherapy, including the types of drugs, dosage, and treatment schedule, is tailored to the individual patient based on the type of cancer, its stage, and the patient's overall health. Oncologists, the doctors who specialize in cancer treatment, carefully monitor patients throughout their chemotherapy to manage side effects and adjust treatment as necessary.

PRACTICAL WAY TO DEAL WITH WEIGHT GAIN DURING CANCER TREATMENT

1. Monitor Your Diet

- **Balanced Meals:** Focus on a balanced diet rich in vegetables, fruits, lean proteins, and whole grains.

- **Portion Control:** Be mindful to not overeat and use smaller plates to watch the quantity of food you consume.

- Healthy Snacking: Choose healthy snacks like nuts, yogurt, and fruits instead of high-calorie, sugary options.

2. Stay Physically Active

- **Regular Exercise:** Incorporate regular physical activity, such as walking, swimming, or yoga. Aim for at least 30 minutes a day, most days of the week.

- **Strength Training:** Include strength training exercises to build muscle mass and boost metabolism.

3. Hydrate Properly

- **Water Intake:** Drink plenty of water to stay hydrated and help control appetite.

- **Limit Sugary Drinks:** Avoid sugary beverages and opt for water, herbal teas, or other low-calorie drinks.

4. Mindful Eating

- **Eat Slowly:** Take your time to eat and savor your food, which can help you recognize when you're full.

- **Avoid Emotional Eating:** Find alternative ways to cope with stress or emotions, such as talking to a friend, practicing relaxation techniques, or engaging in a hobby.

5. Plan and Prepare Meals

- **Meal Prep:** Prepare healthy meals and snacks in advance to avoid the temptation of unhealthy options.

- **Cook at Home:** Cooking at home allows you to control **Ingredients:** and portion sizes better.

6. Seek Professional Guidance

- **Dietitian Consultation:** Work with a registered dietitian who specializes in oncology nutrition to develop a personalized eating plan.

- **Support Groups:** Join a support group to share experiences and tips with others who are facing similar challenges.

7. Medication Management

- **Review Medications:** Some medications can cause weight gain. Discuss with your healthcare provider if this is a concern, as they may adjust your treatment plan.

ANTI-INFLAMMATORY FOODS TO AVOID DURING AND AFTER CHEMO

While following an anti-inflammatory diet during and after chemotherapy can be beneficial, it's important to avoid certain foods that can increase inflammation and potentially interfere with your treatment. Below are some major foods to avoid:

1. Processed and Red Meats: Bacon, sausages, hot dogs, and processed deli meats often contain high levels of saturated fats, preservatives, and other additives that can promote inflammation.

2. Sugary Foods and Beverages: Sodas, candies, pastries, and sugary cereals contain high sugar and can lead to increased inflammation and may affect immune function.

3. Refined Carbohydrates: White bread, white rice, pastries, and most pre-packaged snack foods can cause spikes in blood sugar levels, leading to increased inflammation.

4. Fried Foods: French fries, fried chicken, and other deep-fried snacks are typically high in unhealthy fats and trans fats, which can exacerbate inflammation.

5. Artificial Trans Fats: Margarine, shortening, and foods made with partially hydrogenated oils are trans fats that are known to increase inflammation and are harmful to heart health.

6. High-Fat Dairy Products: Full-fat milk, cheese, and butter contain saturated fats that can contribute to inflammation.

7. Alcohol: Excessive alcohol consumption can lead to increased inflammation and negatively impact liver function, which is crucial during and after chemotherapy.

8. Excessive Salt: Processed foods, canned soups, and fast food have high salt content and high salt intake can contribute to inflammation and increase the risk of hypertension.

9. Certain Additives and Preservatives: MSG (monosodium glutamate), nitrates, and nitrites are found in processed foods. These additives can trigger inflammatory responses in some people.

HEALTHY FOODS TO EAT DURING AND AFTER CHEMO

1. Fruits and Vegetables: Berries, citrus fruits, leafy greens, carrots, sweet potatoes, and bell peppers. are rich in vitamins, minerals, antioxidants, and fiber, which help boost the immune system and reduce inflammation.

2. Lean Proteins: Chicken, turkey, fish, eggs, tofu, beans, and legumes are essential for tissue repair, muscle maintenance, and immune function. Fish such as mackerel salmon supports the body with omega-3 fatty acids.

3. Whole Grains: Oats, quinoa, brown rice, whole wheat bread, and barley provides long-lasting energy, fiber for digestive health, and important nutrients like B vitamins and magnesium.

4. Healthy Fats: Avocados, nuts, seeds, olive oil, and fatty fish supports brain health, reduce inflammation, and provide essential fatty acids.

5. Dairy or Dairy Alternatives: Low-fat yogurt, kefir, and fortified plant-based milk (almond, soy, or oat milk) are good sources of calcium, vitamin D, and probiotics for gut health.

6. Hydrating Foods and Fluids: Water, herbal teas, broths, and hydrating fruits and vegetables like cucumbers and watermelon helps to maintain hydration and manage side effects like dry mouth and constipation, and support overall bodily functions.

7. High-Fiber Foods: Fruits, vegetables, whole grains, beans, and legumes aids in digestion, prevent constipation, and promote a healthy gut microbiome.

8. Antioxidant-Rich Foods: Blueberries, spinach, nuts, and dark chocolate (in moderation) protects cells from damage, support the immune system, and reduce inflammation.

CHAPTER 2

14-DAY MEAL PLAN

DAY 1

Breakfast: Chicken Pasta Bake

Lunch: Green Veggie Bowl with Chicken & Lemon-Tahini Dressing

Dinner: Blueberry Banana Smoothie

DAY 2

Breakfast: Oatmeal Berry Bowl

Lunch: Baked Eggs in Tomato Sauce with Kale

Dinner: Baked Salmon with Peas and Green Mayo Dressing

DAY 3

Breakfast: Lemon Smoothie

Lunch: Chocolate-Peanut Butter Protein Shake

Dinner: Carrot Cake

DAY 4

Breakfast: Baked Oatmeal

Lunch: Roast Chicken & Sweet Potatoes

Dinner: Blueberry Cream Pie

DAY 5

Breakfast: High Protein Blueberry Smoothie

Lunch: Steamed Broccoli with Cheese Sauce

Dinner: Enchilada Power Bowls with Spicy Tofu

DAY 6

Breakfast: Coconut Banana Muffins

Lunch: Chilled Prawn Pasta

Dinner: Chicken Rice Soup

DAY 7

Breakfast: Veggie Soup

Lunch: Lentil Stew

Dinner: Easy Edamame-Pea Dip

DAY 8

Breakfast: Fruit Popsicles

Lunch: Banana Cream Pie

Dinner: Mac & Cheese with Collards

DAY 9

Breakfast: Smoothie Bowl

Lunch: Butternut Squash Soup

Dinner: Chocolate Espresso Mousse

DAY 10

Breakfast: Muffin Tin Eggs

Lunch: Turkey Black Bean Chili

Dinner: Avocado Egg Salad Sandwiches

DAY 11

Breakfast: Chicken Pasta Bake

Lunch: Green Veggie Bowl with Chicken & Lemon-Tahini Dressing

Dinner: Blueberry Banana Smoothie

DAY 12

Breakfast: Oatmeal Berry Bowl

Lunch: Baked Eggs in Tomato Sauce with Kale

Dinner: Baked Salmon with Peas and Green Mayo Dressing

DAY 13

Breakfast: Lemon Smoothie

Lunch: Chocolate-Peanut Butter Protein Shake

Dinner: Carrot Cake

DAY 14

Breakfast: Baked Oatmeal

Lunch: Roast Chicken & Sweet Potatoes

Dinner: Blueberry Cream Pie

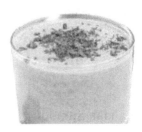

CHAPTER 3

NUTRITIOUS RECIPES FOR NEWLY DIAGNOSED CANCER PATIENTS ON CHEMOTHERAPY

BREAKFAST

Oatmeal Berry Bowl

Preparation Time: 10 minutes

Serves: 1

Calories: 250mg **Carbs:** 45g **Protein:** 7g **Fat:** 6g **Fiber:** 8g **Sodium:** 25mg

Ingredients:

1/2 cup gluten-free rolled oats

1 cup unsweetened almond milk

1/2 cup mixed berries (blueberries, strawberries, raspberries)

1 tablespoon chia seeds

1 tablespoon almond butter

1 teaspoon maple syrup (optional)

1/4 teaspoon ground cinnamon

1/2 teaspoon vanilla extract

1 tablespoon chopped almonds

Method of Preparation:

1. Combine the oats and almond milk in a small saucepan.

2. Bring to a gentle boil over medium heat, then reduce to a simmer.

3. Cook for about 5 minutes, stirring occasionally, until the oats are soft and the mixture turns thick.

4. Stir in the chia seeds, almond butter, maple syrup (if using), cinnamon, and vanilla extract.

5. Continue to cook for another 2-3 minutes, until everything is well combined and heated through.

6. Pour the oatmeal into a bowl.

7. Top with mixed berries and chopped almonds.

8. Serve immediately and enjoy a nutritious, anti-inflammatory breakfast.

Lemon Smoothie

Preparation Time: 5 minutes

Serves: 1

Calories: 180mg **Carbs:** 35g **Protein:** 6g **Fat:** 3g **Fiber:** 6g **Sodium:** 50mg

Ingredients:

1 cup unsweetened almond milk

1/2 cup plain Greek yogurt (dairy-free option available)

1 medium banana

1 tablespoon fresh lemon juice

1 teaspoon lemon zest

1 tablespoon chia seeds

1 teaspoon honey or maple syrup (optional)

1/2 cup ice cubes

Method of Preparation:

1. Gather all Ingredients and ensure the banana is peeled.

2. Place almond milk, Greek yogurt, banana, lemon juice, lemon zest, chia seeds, and honey (if using) in a blender.

3. Add in ice cubes.

4. Blend on high until smooth and creamy, about 1-2 minutes.

5. Pour into a glass and serve immediately.

Baked Oatmeal

Preparation Time: 45 minutes

Serves: 6

Calories: 220mg **Carbs:** 38g **Protein:** 6g **Fat:** 6g **Fiber:** 6g **Sodium:** 30mg

Ingredients:

2 cups gluten-free rolled oats

1/2 cup chopped nuts (almonds or walnuts)

1 teaspoon baking powder

1 teaspoon ground cinnamon

1/4 teaspoon ground nutmeg

1/4 teaspoon turmeric (anti-inflammatory)

2 cups unsweetened almond milk

1/4 cup pure maple syrup

2 tablespoons chia seeds mixed with 6 tablespoons water (egg substitute)

2 teaspoons vanilla extract

1 large apple, diced

1/2 cup blueberries

Method of Preparation:

1. Preheat your oven to 375°F (190°C).
2. Grease a 9x9-inch baking dish with a small amount of oil or non-stick spray.
3. In a large bowl, add oats, chopped nuts, baking powder, cinnamon, nutmeg, and turmeric.
4. In another bowl, whisk together almond milk, maple syrup, chia seed mixture, and vanilla extract.
5. Pour the wet ingredients into the dry ingredients and mix well.
6. Fold in the diced apple and blueberries.

7. Pour the mixture into the prepared baking dish.

8. Bake for 35 minutes, or until the top is golden and the oatmeal is set.

9. Let cool slightly before serving.

10. Cut into squares and enjoy a warm, hearty breakfast or snack.

High Protein Blueberry Smoothie

Preparation Time: 5 minutes

Serves: 1

Calories: 250mg **Carbs:** 35g **Protein:** 20g **Fat:** 5g **Fiber:** 7g **Sodium:** 50mg

Ingredients:

1 cup unsweetened almond milk

1/2 cup frozen blueberries

1/2 banana

1 scoop plant-based protein powder (unflavored or vanilla)

1 tablespoon almond butter

1 tablespoon chia seeds

1 teaspoon pure maple syrup (optional)

1/2 cup ice cubes

Method of Preparation:

1. Peel the banana.
2. In a blender, place almond milk, frozen blueberries, banana, protein powder, almond butter, chia seeds, and maple syrup (if using).
3. Add ice cubes.
4. Blend smoothly on high until creamy, about 1-2 minutes.
5. Pour into a glass and serve immediately.

Coconut Banana Muffins

Preparation Time: 40 minutes

Serves: 12

Calories: 150mg **Carbs:** 25g **Protein:** 3g **Fat:** 5g **Fiber:** 3g **Sodium:** 20mg

Ingredients:

1 1/2 cups gluten-free oat flour

1/2 cup shredded unsweetened coconut

1 teaspoon baking soda

1/2 teaspoon baking powder

1/4 teaspoon ground cinnamon

1/4 teaspoon ground nutmeg

3 medium ripe bananas, mashed

1/4 cup coconut oil, melted

1/4 cup pure maple syrup

2 tablespoons chia seeds mixed with 6 tablespoons water (egg substitute)

1 teaspoon vanilla extract

Method of Preparation:

1. Preheat your oven to 350°F (175°C).
2. Line a 12-cup muffin tin with paper liners or grease with a small amount of coconut oil.
3. Whisk together the oat flour, shredded coconut, baking soda, baking powder, cinnamon, and nutmeg in a large bowl.

4. Mix the mashed bananas, melted coconut oil, maple syrup, chia seed mixture, and vanilla extract in another bowl until well combined.
5. Pour the wet ingredients into the dry Ingredients and stir until just combined.
6. Divide the batter evenly among the 12 muffin cups.
7. Bake: Bake for 20-25 minutes, or until a toothpick inserted into the center of a muffin comes out clean.
8. Let the muffins cool in the tin for 5 minutes, then transfer to a wire rack to cool completely.
9. Enjoy!

Veggie Soup

Preparation Time: 60 minutes

Serves: 6

Calories: 120mg **Carbs:** 25g **Protein:** 4g **Fat:** 2g **Fiber:** 7g **Sodium:** 50mg

Ingredients:

2 tablespoons olive oil

1 large onion, chopped

2 cloves garlic, minced

3 medium carrots, chopped

2 celery stalks, chopped

1 large zucchini, chopped

1 red bell pepper, chopped

1 cup green beans, chopped

1 can (14.5 oz) diced tomatoes, no salt added

6 cups low-sodium vegetable broth

1 teaspoon dried thyme

1 teaspoon dried basil

1/2 teaspoon ground turmeric

1/4 teaspoon ground black pepper

1 cup kale, chopped

1/4 cup chopped fresh parsley

Method of Preparation:

1. In a large pot, heat olive oil over medium heat.

2. Add the onion and garlic, sauté until softened, about 5 minutes.

3. Add the carrots, celery, zucchini, bell pepper, and green beans.

4. Cook for another 5 minutes, stirring occasionally.

5. Stir in the diced tomatoes, vegetable broth, thyme, basil, turmeric, and black pepper.

6. Bring the mixture to a boil, then reduce the heat and simmer for 25-30 minutes, or until the vegetables are tender.

7. Stir in the kale and cook for another 5 minutes.

8. Remove from heat, stir in the fresh parsley, and serve hot.

Fruit Popsicles

Preparation Time: 10 minutes

Freezing Time: 4 hours

Serves:8

Calories: 60mg **Carbs:** 15g **Protein:** 0.5g **Fat:** 0.5g
Fiber: 2g **Sodium:** 5mg

Ingredients:

2 cups mixed fresh or frozen fruit (strawberries, blueberries, mango, etc.)

1 cup unsweetened coconut water

1 tablespoon pure maple syrup (optional)

1 teaspoon fresh lemon juice

Method of Preparation:

1. In a blender, place the mixed fruit, coconut water, maple syrup (if using), and lemon juice.

2. Blend until smooth.

3. Pour the mixture into popsicle molds, leaving a little space at the top for expansion.

4. Place the sticks in the molds.

5. Freeze for at least 4 hours, or until completely solid.

6. To release the popsicles, run warm water over the outside of the molds for a few seconds.

7. Serve immediately and enjoy a refreshing treat.

Smoothie Bowl

Preparation Time: 10 minutes

Serves : 1

Calories: 300mg **Carbs:** 45g **Protein:** 10g **Fat:** 10g
Fiber: 9g **Sodium:** 50mg

Ingredients:

1 cup frozen mixed berries (blueberries, strawberries, raspberries)

1 medium banana

1/2 cup unsweetened almond milk

1/4 cup plain Greek yogurt (dairy-free option available)

1 tablespoon chia seeds

1 tablespoon almond butter

1 teaspoon pure maple syrup (optional)

1/2 teaspoon vanilla extract

Toppings:

1/4 cup sliced fresh fruit (e.g., strawberries, kiwi)

1 tablespoon granola (gluten-free)

1 tablespoon shredded unsweetened coconut

1 tablespoon chia seeds

1 tablespoon chopped nuts (almonds, walnuts)

Method of Preparation:

1. In a blender, combine the frozen mixed berries, banana, almond milk, Greek yogurt, chia seeds, almond butter, maple syrup (if using), and vanilla extract.
2. Blend until smooth and creamy.
3. Pour the smoothie mixture into a bowl.
4. Top with sliced fresh fruit, granola, shredded coconut, chia seeds, and chopped nuts.
5. Serve immediately and enjoy a nutrient-rich breakfast or snack.

Muffin Tin Eggs

Preparation Time: 30 minutes

Serves: 12

Calories: 70mg **Carbs:** 1g **Protein:** 6g **Fat:** 5g **Fiber:** 0.5g **Sodium:** 60mg

Ingredients:

8 large eggs

1/4 cup unsweetened almond milk

1/2 cup diced bell peppers (any color)

1/2 cup chopped spinach

1/4 cup diced onion

1/4 cup chopped tomatoes

1/4 teaspoon ground black pepper

1/4 teaspoon turmeric (anti-inflammatory)

1/4 teaspoon dried basil

1/4 teaspoon dried thyme

Method of Preparation:

1. Preheat your oven to 350°F (175°C).
2. Grease a 12-cup muffin tin with a small amount of olive oil or non-stick spray.
3. In a large bowl, whisk together the eggs and almond milk until well combined.
4. Stir in the diced bell peppers, chopped spinach, diced onion, chopped tomatoes, black pepper, turmeric, basil, and thyme.

5. Pour the egg mixture evenly into the 12 muffin cups.

6. Bake for 20 minutes, or until the eggs are set and slightly golden on top.

7. Let cool for a few minutes before removing from the tin.

8. Serve warm or at room temperature. These can be stored in the refrigerator for up to 3 days.

Chicken Pasta Bake

Preparation Time: 60 minutes

Serves: 6

Calories: 350mg **Carbs:** 45g **Protein:** 25g **Fat:** 10g **Fiber:** 5g **Sodium:** 40mg

Ingredients:

8 oz gluten-free pasta (penne or fusilli)

1 tablespoon olive oil

2 cups cooked, shredded chicken breast

1 large onion, diced

2 cloves garlic, minced

1 red bell pepper, diced

1 zucchini, diced

1 cup baby spinach, chopped

1 can (14.5 oz) diced tomatoes, no salt added

1 teaspoon dried basil

1 teaspoon dried oregano

1/4 teaspoon ground black pepper

1/4 teaspoon turmeric (anti-inflammatory)

1 cup shredded dairy-free mozzarella cheese (or regular, if preferred)

Method of Preparation:

1. Preheat oven to 375°F (190°C).
2. Cook pasta according to package instructions until al dente.
3. Drain and set aside.
4. In a large pan, heat olive oil over medium heat.

5. Add the onion and garlic, sauté for 5 minutes until softened.

6. Add the bell pepper and zucchini, cook for another 5 minutes until vegetables are tender.

7. Stir in the cooked chicken, diced tomatoes, basil, oregano, black pepper, and turmeric.

8. Cook for 5 more minutes, then add the chopped spinach and cooked pasta.

9. Mix well to combine.

10. Transfer the mixture to a greased 9x13-inch baking dish.

11. Sprinkle the shredded cheese evenly over the top.

12. Bake for 20-25 minutes, or until the cheese is melted and bubbly.

13. Let cool for a few minutes before serving.

14. Enjoy a comforting, nutritious meal.

LUNCH

Green Veggie Bowl with Chicken & Lemon-Tahini Dressing

Preparation Time: 40 minutes

Serves: 2

Calories: 400mg **Carbs:** 20g **Protein:** 30g **Fat:** 20g
Fiber: 8g **Sodium:** 150mg

Ingredients:

For the Bowl:

2 boneless, skinless chicken breasts

2 cups mixed greens (spinach, kale, arugula)

1 cup broccoli florets

1 cup snap peas, trimmed

1/2 avocado, sliced

1/4 cup pumpkin seeds (pepitas), toasted

1 tablespoon olive oil

A pinch of salt and pepper

For the Lemon-Tahini Dressing:

2 tablespoons tahini

2 tablespoons fresh lemon juice

1 tablespoon water

1 clove garlic, minced

A pinch of salt and pepper

Method of Preparation:

1. Preheat your oven to 400°F (200°C).
2. Line a baking sheet with parchment paper.
3. Season chicken breasts with salt, pepper, and a drizzle of olive oil.
4. Place on the prepared baking sheet and roast for 20 minutes, or until cooked through.
5. Let them rest for a few minutes before slicing.
6. While the chicken is cooking, steam broccoli florets and snap peas until tender, about 5 minutes.
7. Drain and set aside.
8. In a small bowl, whisk together tahini, lemon juice, water, minced garlic, salt, and pepper until smooth.
9. Divide mixed greens between two bowls.
10. Top with steamed broccoli, snap peas, sliced avocado, and sliced roasted chicken.
11. Sprinkle with toasted pumpkin seeds.
12. Drizzle lemon-tahini dressing over the bowls.

13. Serve immediately and enjoy this vibrant and nutritious meal.

Baked Eggs in Tomato Sauce with Kale

Preparation Time: 40 minutes

Serves: 4

Calories: 200mg **Carbs:** 15g **Protein:** 10g **Fat:** 10g **Fiber:** 5g **Sodium:** 60mg

Ingredients:

2 tablespoons olive oil

1 onion, finely chopped

2 cloves garlic, minced

1 can (14.5 oz) diced tomatoes, no salt added

1 teaspoon dried oregano

1/2 teaspoon dried basil

A pinch of salt and pepper

4 large eggs

2 cups kale, chopped

Method of Preparation:

1. Preheat your oven to 375°F (190°C).
2. In an oven-safe pan, heat olive oil over medium heat.
3. Add chopped onion and minced garlic, sauté until softened, about 5 minutes.
4. Stir in diced tomatoes (with their juices), dried oregano, dried basil, salt, and pepper.
5. Simmer for 5 minutes.
6. Add chopped kale to the pan and cook until wilted, about 2 minutes.
7. Using a spoon, make four wells in the tomato sauce mixture.
8. Crack an egg into each well.
9. Transfer the pan to the preheated oven and bake for 12-15 minutes, or until the egg whites are set but the yolks are still runny.
10. Remove from oven, let cool for a few minutes, and serve warm.
11. Enjoy with crusty bread or a side salad.

Chocolate-Peanut Butter Protein Shake

Preparation Time: 5 minutes

Serves: 1

Calories: 300mg **Carbs:** 25g **Protein:** 25g **Fat:** 10g
Fiber: 5g **Sodium:** 150mg

Ingredients:

1 cup unsweetened almond milk

1 scoop chocolate protein powder (plant-based)

1 tablespoon natural peanut butter

1 tablespoon cocoa powder

1/2 banana, frozen

1/2 cup ice cubes

Method of Preparation:

1. Add almond milk, chocolate protein powder, peanut butter, cocoa powder, frozen banana, and ice cubes to a blender.

2. Blend smoothly on high speed until creamy.

3. Pour into a glass and enjoy immediately.

4. Optionally, garnish with a sprinkle of cocoa powder or a drizzle of peanut butter.

Roast Chicken & Sweet Potatoes

Preparation Time: 60 minutes

Serves: 4

Calories: 350mg **Carbs:** 30g **Protein:** 25g **Fat:** 15g
Fiber: 5g **Sodium:** 70mg

Ingredients:

4 bone-in, skin-on chicken thighs

2 large sweet potatoes, peeled and cubed

1 tablespoon olive oil

1 teaspoon smoked paprika

1 teaspoon garlic powder

1 teaspoon dried thyme

A pinch of salt and pepper

Fresh parsley, chopped (for garnish)

Method of Preparation:

1. Preheat your oven to 400°F (200°C).
2. Line a baking sheet with parchment paper.
3. Pat chicken thighs dry with paper towels.
4. Rub with olive oil, smoked paprika, garlic powder, dried thyme, salt, and pepper.
5. In a bowl, toss cubed sweet potatoes with olive oil, salt, and pepper until evenly coated.
6. Place seasoned chicken thighs and sweet potatoes on the prepared baking sheet in a single layer.
7. Bake for 35-40 minutes, or until chicken is cooked through and sweet potatoes are tender, flipping sweet potatoes halfway through.
8. Remove from oven, let cool for a few minutes, and serve warm.
9. Garnish with chopped fresh parsley if desired.

Steamed Broccoli with Cheese Sauce

Preparation Time: 25 minutes

Serves: 4

Calories: 150mg **Carbs:** 10g **Protein:** 8g **Fat:** 10g **Fiber:** 4g **Sodium:** 50mg

Ingredients:

For the Steamed Broccoli:

4 cups broccoli florets

Water for steaming

A pinch of salt

For the Cheese Sauce:

1 tablespoon unsalted butter

1 tablespoon gluten-free all-purpose flour

1 cup unsweetened almond milk

1 cup shredded cheddar cheese

A pinch of salt and pepper

Method of Preparation:

1. Place broccoli florets in a steamer basket over boiling water.

2. Cover and steam for 5-7 minutes, or until tender but still crisp.

3. Remove from heat and set aside.

4. In a small saucepan, melt butter over medium heat.

5. Whisk in flour and cook for 1-2 minutes, until lightly golden.

6. Gradually whisk in almond milk until smooth and thickened.

7. Stir in shredded cheddar cheese until melted and creamy.

8. Season with a pinch of salt and pepper.

9. Arrange steamed broccoli on a serving dish and drizzle with cheese sauce.

10. Serve immediately and enjoy with any choice of main dish.

Chilled Prawn Pasta

Preparation Time: 25 minutes

Serves: 4

Calories: 300mg **Carbs:** 25g **Protein:** 20g **Fat:** 12g
Fiber: 3g **Sodium:** 80mg

Ingredients:

8 oz gluten-free pasta (spaghetti or penne)

1 lb. cooked prawns (shrimp), peeled and deveined

1 cup cherry tomatoes, halved

1/2 cup diced cucumber

1/4 cup chopped fresh parsley

2 tablespoons extra virgin olive oil

2 tablespoons fresh lemon juice

2 cloves garlic, minced

A pinch of salt and pepper

Method of Preparation:

1. Cook gluten-free pasta according to package instructions until al dente.
2. Drain and rinse under cold water to cool.
3. Transfer to a large mixing bowl.
4. In a small bowl, whisk together extra virgin olive oil, lemon juice, minced garlic, salt, and pepper.

5. Add cooked prawns, halved cherry tomatoes, diced cucumber, and chopped parsley to the bowl with the cooked pasta.

6. Pour the dressing over the pasta and toss gently to combine, ensuring everything is evenly coated.

7. Cover the bowl with plastic wrap and chill in the refrigerator for at least 1 hour to allow flavors to meld.

8. Remove from refrigerator, toss once more, and serve chilled as a refreshing and satisfying pasta salad.

Lentil Stew

Preparation Time: 60 minutes

Serves: 6

Calories: 250mg **Carbs:** 40g **Protein:** 15g **Fat:** 2g **Fiber:** 10g **Sodium:** 50mg

Ingredients:

1 cup dried green or brown lentils, rinsed and drained

4 cups low-sodium vegetable broth

1 onion, diced

2 carrots, diced

2 celery stalks, diced

2 cloves garlic, minced

1 can (14.5 oz) diced tomatoes, no salt added

1 teaspoon ground cumin

1 teaspoon paprika

1/2 teaspoon dried thyme

A pinch of salt and pepper

Fresh parsley, chopped (for garnish)

Method of Preparation:

1. In a large pot, combine rinsed lentils and vegetable broth.
2. Bring to a boil, then reduce heat to low and simmer for 20 minutes.
3. In a separate pan, heat olive oil over medium heat.
4. Add diced onion, carrots, and celery.
5. Sauté until softened, about 5 minutes.

6. Add minced garlic and cook for an additional minute.

7. Add sautéed vegetables, diced tomatoes (with their juices), ground cumin, paprika, dried thyme, salt, and pepper to the pot with the cooked lentils.

8. Stir to combine.

9. Continue to simmer the stew for an additional 20-25 minutes, stirring occasionally, until lentils and vegetables are tender and flavors are well combined.

10. Ladle into bowls, garnish with chopped fresh parsley if desired, and serve hot.

Banana Cream Pie

Preparation Time: 40 minutes

Serves: 8

Calories: 300mg **Carbs:** 35g **Protein:** 4g **Fat:** 15g **Fiber:** 2g **Sodium:** 20mg

Ingredients:

For the Crust:

1 1/2 cups gluten-free graham cracker crumbs

6 tablespoons unsalted butter, melted

For the Filling:

3 ripe bananas, sliced

1/2 cup granulated sugar

1/4 cup cornstarch

2 cups unsweetened almond milk

3 large egg yolks

1 teaspoon vanilla extract

For the Topping:

1 cup whipped cream (dairy or dairy-free)

Sliced bananas for garnish

Method of Preparation:

1. In a bowl, mix together gluten-free graham cracker crumbs and melted butter until well combined.
2. Press mixture into the bottom and up the sides of a 9-inch pie dish.
3. Chill in the refrigerator while preparing the filling.

4. In a saucepan, combine sliced bananas, granulated sugar, cornstarch, almond milk, and egg yolks.

5. Cook over medium heat, stirring constantly, until mixture thickens, about 5-7 minutes.

6. Remove from heat and stir in vanilla extract.

7. Pour banana filling into the prepared crust.

8. Smooth the top with a spatula.

9. Chill in the refrigerator for at least 4 hours, or until set.

10. Before serving, spread whipped cream over the chilled pie.

11. Garnish with sliced bananas.

12. Slice and serve cold.

13. Enjoy this creamy and delicious banana cream pie as a delightful dessert.

Butternut Squash Soup

Preparation Time: 45 minutes

Serves: 6

Calories: 200mg **Carbs:** 25g **Protein:** 3g **Fat:** 10g **Fiber:** 5g **Sodium:** 50mg

Ingredients:

1 medium butternut squash, peeled, seeded, and diced

1 onion, chopped

2 cloves garlic, minced

2 carrots, chopped

2 stalks celery, chopped

4 cups low-sodium vegetable broth

1 teaspoon dried thyme

1/2 teaspoon ground nutmeg

A pinch of salt and pepper

2 tablespoons olive oil

Method of Preparation:

1. In a large pot, heat olive oil over medium heat.
2. Add chopped onion, minced garlic, chopped carrots, and chopped celery.
3. Sauté until vegetables are softened, about 5 minutes.

4. Add diced butternut squash to the pot and cook for another 5 minutes, stirring occasionally.
5. Pour in vegetable broth, dried thyme, ground nutmeg, salt, and pepper.
6. Bring to a boil, then reduce heat and simmer for 20 minutes, or until squash is tender.
7. Use an immersion blender to puree the soup until smooth.
8. Alternatively, carefully transfer soup to a blender and blend in batches until smooth.
9. Taste and adjust seasoning as needed with salt and pepper.
10. Ladle into bowls and serve hot.
11. Optionally, garnish with a drizzle of olive oil or a sprinkle of fresh thyme.

Turkey Black Bean Chili

Preparation Time: 1 hour, 15 minutes

Serves: 6

Calories: 300mg **Carbs:** 25g **Protein:** 25g **Fat:** 10g
Fiber: 8g **Sodium:** 50mg

Ingredients:

1 lb. ground turkey

1 onion, chopped

2 cloves garlic, minced

1 bell pepper, chopped

1 can (14.5 oz) diced tomatoes, no salt added

2 cups low-sodium chicken broth

1 can (15 oz) black beans, rinsed and drained

1 cup frozen corn kernels

2 tablespoons chili powder

1 teaspoon ground cumin

1/2 teaspoon paprika

A pinch of salt and pepper

2 tablespoons olive oil

Method of Preparation:

1. In a large pot, heat olive oil over medium heat.

2. Add ground turkey and cook until browned, breaking it up with a spoon, about 5-7 minutes.
3. Add chopped onion, minced garlic, and chopped bell pepper to the pot.
4. Sauté until vegetables are softened, about 5 minutes.
5. Stir in diced tomatoes (with their juices), low-sodium chicken broth, black beans, frozen corn kernels, chili powder, ground cumin, paprika, salt, and pepper.
6. Bring chili to a boil, then reduce heat and simmer for 45 minutes to 1 hour, stirring occasionally, until flavors are well combined and chili has thickened.
7. Ladle into bowls and serve hot.

DINNER

Avocado Egg Salad Sandwiches

Preparation Time: 25 minutes

Serves: 4

Calories: 300mg **Carbs:** 20g **Protein:** 12g **Fat:** 20g
Fiber: 8g **Sodium:** 80mg

Ingredients:

6 hard-boiled eggs, peeled and chopped

1 ripe avocado, mashed

2 tablespoons Greek yogurt (or mayo)

1 tablespoon Dijon mustard

1 tablespoon fresh lemon juice

1/4 cup chopped celery

1/4 cup chopped red onion

A pinch of salt and pepper

8 slices whole grain bread

Lettuce leaves and tomato slices for serving

Method of Preparation:

1. In a large bowl, place chopped hard-boiled eggs, mashed avocado, Greek yogurt (or mayo), Dijon mustard, lemon juice, chopped celery, and chopped red onion.
2. Mix well to combine.
3. Season with a pinch of salt and pepper.

4. Spread a generous amount of avocado egg salad onto one slice of bread.

5. Top with lettuce leaves, tomato slices, and another slice of bread.

6. Repeat with remaining ingredients to make 4 sandwiches.

7. Serve immediately or wrap tightly in plastic wrap for later.

8. Enjoy these flavorful and satisfying avocado egg salad sandwiches!

Chocolate Espresso Mousse

Preparation Time: 15 minutes

Serves: 4

Calories: 250mg **Carbs:** 20g **Protein:** 5g **Fat:** 18g **Fiber:** 4g **Sodium:** 20mg

Ingredients:

2 ripe avocados, peeled and pitted

1/4 cup unsweetened cocoa powder

1/4 cup maple syrup or honey

1 teaspoon instant espresso powder

1 teaspoon vanilla extract

Pinch of salt

Fresh berries for garnish (optional)

Method of Preparation:

1. Blend: In a food processor or blender, combine peeled and pitted avocados, unsweetened cocoa powder, maple syrup (or honey), instant espresso powder, vanilla extract, and a pinch of salt. Blend until smooth and creamy.
2. Chill: Transfer the chocolate espresso mousse to serving glasses or bowls. Cover and chill in the refrigerator for at least 2 hours, or until firm.
3. Serve: Before serving, garnish with fresh berries if desired. Enjoy this indulgent and creamy chocolate espresso mousse as a delightful dessert!

Mac & Cheese with Collards

Preparation Time: 40 minutes

Serves: 6

Calories: 350mg **Carbs:** 40g **Protein:** 15g **Fat:** 15g

Fiber: 5g **Sodium:** 450mg

Ingredients:

8 oz elbow macaroni (gluten-free if desired)

2 cups chopped collard greens; stems removed

2 tablespoons unsalted butter

2 tablespoons gluten-free all-purpose flour

2 cups unsweetened almond milk

2 cups shredded sharp cheddar cheese

A pinch of salt and pepper

1/4 cup gluten-free breadcrumbs (optional)

Method of Preparation:

1. Cook Pasta: Cook elbow macaroni according to package instructions until al dente. Drain and set aside.

2. Prepare Collards: In a pot of boiling water, blanch chopped collard greens for 2-3 minutes until tender. Drain and set aside.

3. Make Cheese Sauce: In a large pan, melt unsalted butter over medium heat. Whisk in gluten-free all-purpose flour and cook for 1-2 minutes until lightly golden. Gradually whisk in unsweetened almond milk until smooth and thickened. Stir in shredded sharp cheddar cheese until melted and creamy. Season with A pinch of salt and pepper.

4. Combine: Add cooked elbow macaroni and blanched collard greens to the cheese sauce. Stir until well combined.

5. Bake: Transfer the mac and cheese mixture to a baking dish. If desired, sprinkle gluten-free breadcrumbs over the top for a crunchy topping.

6. Bake: Bake in a preheated oven at 350°F (175°C) for 15-20 minutes until bubbly and golden on top.

7. Serve: Remove from oven and let cool for a few minutes before serving. Enjoy this comforting and nutritious mac & cheese with collards as a satisfying meal!

Easy Edamame-Pea Dip

Preparation Time: 10 minutes

Serves: 6

Calories: 100mg **Carbs:** 8g **Protein:** 6g **Fat:** 6g **Fiber:** 3g **Sodium:** 150mg

Ingredients:

1 cup shelled edamame, cooked

1 cup frozen peas, thawed

2 tablespoons tahini

2 tablespoons fresh lemon juice

1 clove garlic, minced

2 tablespoons extra virgin olive oil

A pinch of salt and pepper

Fresh herbs for garnish (optional)

Method of Preparation:

1. Blend: In a food processor or blender, combine cooked shelled edamame, thawed frozen peas, tahini, fresh lemon juice, minced garlic, extra virgin olive oil, salt, and pepper.

2. Blend until Smooth: Blend until smooth and creamy, scraping down the sides as needed.

3. Adjust Consistency: If the dip is too thick, add a splash of water or more olive oil to reach your desired consistency.

4. Season to Taste: Taste and adjust seasoning with salt and pepper as needed.

5. Serve: Transfer the dip to a serving bowl. Garnish with fresh herbs if desired. Serve with sliced vegetables, crackers, or pita bread for dipping. Enjoy this nutritious and flavorful edamame-pea dip!

Chicken Rice Soup

Preparation Time: 45 minutes

Serves: 4

Calories: 250mg **Carbs:** 30g **Protein:** 20g **Fat:** 6g **Fiber:** 3g **Sodium:** 400mg

Ingredients:

1 tablespoon olive oil

1 onion, diced

2 carrots, diced

2 celery stalks, diced

2 cloves garlic, minced

6 cups low-sodium chicken broth

1 cup cooked chicken breast, shredded

1 cup cooked rice

1 teaspoon dried thyme

A pinch of salt and pepper

Fresh parsley for garnish (optional)

Method of Preparation:

1. Sauté Vegetables: In a large pot, heat olive oil over medium heat. Add diced onion, carrots, and celery. Sauté until vegetables are softened, about 5 minutes.
2. Add Garlic: Add minced garlic and cook for another minute until fragrant.
3. Add Broth: Pour in low-sodium chicken broth and bring to a simmer.

4. Add Chicken and Rice: Stir in shredded cooked chicken breast and cooked rice.

5. Season: Season with dried thyme, salt, and pepper to taste.

6. Simmer: Simmer soup for 15-20 minutes to allow flavors to meld.

7. Serve: Ladle into bowls, garnish with fresh parsley if desired, and serve hot. Enjoy this comforting and nourishing chicken rice soup!

Enchilada Power Bowls with Spicy Tofu

Preparation Time: 45 minutes

Serves: 4

Calories: 400mg **Carbs:** 40g **Protein:** 20g **Fat:** 18g **Fiber:** 10g **Sodium:** 600mg

Ingredients:

For the Spicy Tofu:

14 oz extra firm tofu, pressed and cubed

2 tablespoons soy sauce (or tamari for gluten-free)

1 tablespoon sriracha sauce

1 tablespoon maple syrup

1 tablespoon olive oil

For the Bowls:

2 cups cooked quinoa

1 can (15 oz) black beans, rinsed and drained

1 cup corn kernels, fresh or frozen

1 bell pepper, diced

1 avocado, sliced

1/4 cup chopped fresh cilantro

Lime wedges for serving

For the Enchilada Sauce:

1 can (15 oz) tomato sauce

1 tablespoon chili powder

1 teaspoon ground cumin

1 teaspoon garlic powder

A pinch of salt and pepper

Method of Preparation:

1. Prepare Spicy Tofu: In a bowl, whisk together soy sauce, sriracha sauce, maple syrup, and olive oil. Add cubed tofu and toss to coat. Let marinate for 10-15 minutes.

2. Cook Tofu: Heat a non-stick pan over medium-high heat. Add marinated tofu and cook for 5-7 minutes, stirring occasionally, until tofu is browned and crispy on all sides. Remove from heat and set aside.

3. Prepare Enchilada Sauce: In a small saucepan, combine tomato sauce, chili powder, ground cumin, garlic powder, salt, and pepper. Bring to a simmer and cook for 5 minutes, stirring occasionally, until sauce is slightly thickened. Remove from heat and set aside.

4. Assemble Bowls: Divide cooked quinoa among serving bowls. Top with black beans, corn kernels, diced bell pepper, sliced avocado, and spicy tofu. Drizzle with enchilada sauce and sprinkle with chopped cilantro. Serve with lime wedges on the side.

5. Serve: Serve immediately, and enjoy these flavorful and nutritious enchilada power bowls!

Blueberry Cream Pie

Preparation Time: 30 minutes

Serves: 8

Calories: 350mg **Carbs:** 40g **Protein:** 4g **Fat:** 20g **Fiber:** 3g **Sodium:** 150mg

Ingredients:

For the Crust:

1 1/2 cups gluten-free graham cracker crumbs

6 tablespoons unsalted butter, melted

For the Filling:

1 1/2 cups fresh blueberries

1/4 cup granulated sugar

1 tablespoon cornstarch

1 cup heavy cream

8 oz cream cheese, softened

1/2 cup powdered sugar

1 teaspoon vanilla extract

Zest of 1 lemon

Method of Preparation:

1. Prepare Crust: In a bowl, mix together gluten-free graham cracker crumbs and melted butter until well combined. Press mixture into the bottom and up the sides of a 9-inch pie dish. Chill in the refrigerator while preparing the filling.

2. Prepare Filling: In a small saucepan, combine fresh blueberries, granulated sugar, and cornstarch. Cook over medium heat, stirring constantly, until mixture thickens and blueberries burst, about 5-7 minutes. Remove from heat and let cool completely.

3. Whip Cream: In a separate bowl, whip heavy cream until stiff peaks form. Set aside.

4. Prepare Cream Cheese Mixture: In another bowl, beat cream cheese, powdered sugar, vanilla extract, and lemon zest until smooth and creamy.

5. Combine Fillings: Gently fold whipped cream into the cream cheese mixture until well combined.

Spread half of the cream cheese mixture onto the chilled crust.

6. Add Blueberry Filling: Spoon cooled blueberry mixture over the cream cheese layer. Top with the remaining cream cheese mixture, spreading evenly.

7. Chill: Cover and chill the pie in the refrigerator for at least 4 hours, or until set.

8. Serve: Slice and serve cold. Enjoy this creamy and fruity blueberry cream pie as a delightful dessert!

Carrot Cake

Preparation Time: 60 minutes

Serves: 12

Calories: 320mg **Carbs:** 45g **Protein:** 3g **Fat:** 15g **Fiber:** 2g **Sodium:** 200mg

Ingredients:

For the Cake:

2 cups gluten-free all-purpose flour

1 1/2 cups granulated sugar

1 teaspoon baking powder

1/2 teaspoon baking soda

1/2 teaspoon salt

1 teaspoon ground cinnamon

1/2 teaspoon ground nutmeg

1/2 teaspoon ground ginger

3 large eggs

1 cup vegetable oil

2 cups grated carrots

1/2 cup chopped walnuts (optional)

1/2 cup crushed pineapple, drained

For the Cream Cheese Frosting:

8 oz cream cheese, softened

1/2 cup unsalted butter, softened

2 cups powdered sugar

1 teaspoon vanilla extract

Method of Preparation:

1. Preheat your oven to 350°F (175°C). Grease and flour two 9-inch round cake pans.

2. In a large mixing bowl, whisk together gluten-free all-purpose flour, granulated sugar, baking powder, baking soda, salt, ground cinnamon, ground nutmeg, and ground ginger.

3. Add eggs and vegetable oil to the dry ingredients.

4. Mix until well combined.

5. Fold in grated carrots, chopped walnuts (if using), and crushed pineapple until evenly distributed in the batter.

6. Divide the batter evenly between the prepared cake pans. Bake in the preheated oven for 25-30 minutes, or until a toothpick inserted into the center comes out clean.

7. Allow the cakes to cool in the pans for 10 minutes, then transfer them to wire racks to cool completely.

8. In a mixing bowl, beat softened cream cheese and unsalted butter until smooth and creamy. Gradually add powdered sugar and vanilla extract, beating until frosting is light and fluffy.

9. Once the cakes are completely cool, spread a layer of cream cheese frosting on top of one cake layer. Place the second cake layer on top and frost the top and sides of the cake with the remaining frosting.

10. Slice and serve your delicious carrot cake. Enjoy!

Baked Salmon with Peas and Green Mayo Dressing

Preparation Time: 30 minutes

Serves: 4

Calories: 350mg **Carbs:** 10g **Protein:** 25g **Fat:** 20g **Fiber:** 3g **Sodium:** 350mg

Ingredients:

For the Salmon:

4 salmon fillets

2 tablespoons olive oil

A pinch of salt and pepper

For the Peas:

2 cups frozen peas, thawed

2 tablespoons unsalted butter

A pinch of salt and pepper

For the Green Mayo Dressing:

1/2 cup mayonnaise

1/4 cup chopped fresh parsley

2 tablespoons chopped fresh dill

1 tablespoon chopped fresh chives

1 tablespoon lemon juice

A pinch of salt and pepper

Method of Preparation:

1. Preheat your oven to 375°F (190°C).
2. Season Salmon: Rub salmon fillets with olive oil and season with salt and pepper.
3. Place salmon fillets on a baking sheet lined with parchment paper. Bake in the preheated oven for 15-20 minutes, or until salmon is cooked through and flakes easily with a fork.
4. In a small saucepan, melt unsalted butter over medium heat. Add thawed peas and cook for 5-7

minutes, or until peas are heated through. Season with A pinch of salt and pepper.

5. In a bowl, combine mayonnaise, chopped fresh parsley, chopped fresh dill, chopped fresh chives, lemon juice, salt, and pepper. Mix until well combined.

6. Serve baked salmon with peas on the side. Drizzle salmon with green mayo dressing or serve it on the side for dipping. Enjoy this flavorful and nutritious dish!

Blueberry Banana Smoothie

Preparation Time: 5 minutes

Serves: 2

Calories: 180mg **Carbs:** 40g **Protein:** 3g **Fat:** 2g **Fiber:** 5g **Sodium:** 10mg

Ingredients:

1 ripe banana

1 cup fresh or frozen blueberries

1/2 cup plain Greek yogurt (or dairy-free alternative)

1/2 cup unsweetened almond milk (or any milk of your choice)

1 tablespoon honey or maple syrup (optional)

Ice cubes (if using fresh blueberries)

Method of Preparation:

1. In a blender, combine ripe banana, fresh or frozen blueberries, plain Greek yogurt, unsweetened almond milk, and honey or maple syrup if using.

2. Blend until smooth and creamy. If using fresh blueberries, add a handful of ice cubes to the blender to chill and thicken the smoothie.

3. If the smoothie is too thick, add more almond milk until you reach your desired consistency. If it's too thin, add more banana or blueberries.

4. Pour the blueberry banana smoothie into glasses and serve immediately. Enjoy this refreshing and nutritious smoothie as a breakfast or snack option!

SALAD

Mediterranean White Bean and Tuna Salad

Preparation Time: 15 minutes

Serves: 4

Calories: 280mg **Carbs:** 25g **Protein:** 22g **Fat:** 10g
Fiber: 7g **Sodium:** 450mg

Ingredients:

2 cans (15 oz each) white beans, drained and rinsed

2 cans (5 oz each) tuna, drained

1 cup cherry tomatoes, halved

1/2 cup cucumber, diced

1/4 cup red onion, thinly sliced

1/4 cup Kalamata olives, pitted and halved

2 tablespoons fresh parsley, chopped

2 tablespoons extra virgin olive oil

1 tablespoon red wine vinegar

A pinch of salt and pepper

1 lemon, sliced (for garnish)

Method of Preparation:

1. In a large mixing bowl, combine the white beans, tuna, cherry tomatoes, cucumber, red onion, Kalamata olives, and chopped parsley.
2. Drizzle the salad with extra virgin olive oil and red wine vinegar. Season with A pinch of salt and pepper.
3. Gently toss the salad until all ingredients are well combined.
4. Divide the salad among serving plates.
5. Garnish with lemon slices.
6. Serve immediately, or refrigerate for up to 1 day before serving. Enjoy this Mediterranean-inspired white bean and tuna salad!

Grilled Fruit Salad

Preparation Time: 15 minutes

Serves: 4

Calories: 150mg **Carbs:** 38g **Protein:** 2g **Fat:** 0.5g **Fiber:** 5g **Sodium:** 5mg

Ingredients:

2 peaches, pitted and sliced

2 nectarines, pitted and sliced

1 cup strawberries, hulled and halved

1 cup pineapple chunks

1 tablespoon honey

1 tablespoon fresh lemon juice

Fresh mint leaves for garnish

Method of Preparation:

1. Preheat a grill or grill pan over medium heat.
2. In a bowl, toss the sliced peaches, nectarines, strawberries, and pineapple chunks with honey and fresh lemon juice until well coated.
3. Grill the fruit for 2-3 minutes on each side, or until lightly charred and caramelized.
4. Remove the grilled fruit from the grill and transfer to a serving platter.

5. Garnish with fresh mint leaves.

6. Serve immediately as a side dish or dessert. Enjoy this flavorful and vibrant grilled fruit salad!

Summer Berry Salad with Herbed Tofu Croutons

Preparation Time: 25 minutes

Serves: 4

Calories: 220mg **Carbs:** 20g **Protein:** 14g **Fat:** 10g **Fiber:** 8g **Sodium:** 350mg

Ingredients:

For the Salad:

6 cups mixed salad greens (such as spinach, arugula, and lettuce)

1 cup strawberries, sliced

1 cup blueberries

1/2 cup raspberries

1/4 cup sliced almonds

1/4 cup crumbled feta cheese (optional)

For the Herbed Tofu Croutons:

8 oz firm tofu, drained and cubed

1 tablespoon olive oil

1 tablespoon fresh herbs (such as parsley, basil, or thyme), chopped

A pinch of salt and pepper

For the Dressing:

2 tablespoons balsamic vinegar

1 tablespoon extra-virgin olive oil

1 teaspoon honey

1 teaspoon Dijon mustard

A pinch of salt and pepper

Method of Preparation:

1. Preheat the oven to 400°F (200°C).

2. In a bowl, toss the cubed tofu with olive oil, chopped fresh herbs, salt, and pepper until evenly coated.

3. Spread the tofu cubes in a single layer on a baking sheet lined with parchment paper.

4. Bake in the preheated oven for 20-25 minutes, or until the tofu is golden and crispy.

5. In a large salad bowl, combine the mixed salad greens, sliced strawberries, blueberries, raspberries, sliced almonds, and crumbled feta cheese (if using).

6. In a small bowl, whisk together balsamic vinegar, extra virgin olive oil, honey, Dijon mustard, salt, and pepper to make the dressing.

7. Drizzle the dressing over the salad and toss gently to coat.

8. Top the salad with the herbed tofu croutons.

9. Serve immediately as a refreshing and nutritious summer berry salad!

Greek Salad with Edamame

Preparation Time: 15 minutes

Serves: 4

Calories: 200mg **Carbs:** 15g **Protein:** 10g **Fat:** 12g **Fiber:** 6g **Sodium:** 300mg

Ingredients:

2 cups mixed salad greens (such as romaine, spinach, and arugula)

1 cup cherry tomatoes, halved

1/2 English cucumber, diced

1/4 cup Kalamata olives, pitted

1/4 cup crumbled feta cheese

1/4 cup shelled edamame beans

2 tablespoons extra virgin olive oil

1 tablespoon red wine vinegar

1 teaspoon dried oregano

A pinch of salt and pepper

Method of Preparation:

1. In a large salad bowl, combine the mixed salad greens, cherry tomatoes, diced cucumber, Kalamata

olives, crumbled feta cheese, and shelled edamame beans.

2. In a small bowl, whisk together the extra virgin olive oil, red wine vinegar, dried oregano, salt, and pepper to make the dressing.

3. Drizzle the dressing over the salad and toss gently to coat all the ingredients.

4. Serve immediately as a refreshing and flavorful Greek salad with edamame! Enjoy as a light meal or side dish.

Chickpea and Veggie Salad

Preparation Time: 15 minutes

Serves: 4

Calories: 250mg **Carbs:** 30g **Protein:** 9g **Fat:** 11g **Fiber:** 9g **Sodium:** 350mg

Ingredients:

2 cups cooked chickpeas (or 1 can, drained and rinsed)

1 cup cherry tomatoes, halved

1/2 English cucumber, diced

1/4 cup red onion, thinly sliced

1/4 cup chopped fresh parsley

1/4 cup crumbled feta cheese (optional)

2 tablespoons extra virgin olive oil

1 tablespoon lemon juice

1 teaspoon Dijon mustard

A pinch of salt and pepper

Method of Preparation:

1. In a large salad bowl, combine the cooked chickpeas, cherry tomatoes, diced cucumber, thinly sliced red onion, chopped fresh parsley, and crumbled feta cheese (if using).

2. In a small bowl, whisk together the extra virgin olive oil, lemon juice, Dijon mustard, salt, and pepper to make the dressing.

3. Drizzle the dressing over the salad and toss gently to coat all the ingredients

4. Serve immediately as a nutritious and satisfying chickpea and veggie salad! Enjoy as a main dish or side dish.

SEAFOOD MAINS

Lemon-Herb Salmon with Caponata & Faro

Preparation Time: 45 minutes

Serves: 4

Calories: 380mg **Carbs:** 40g **Protein:** 28g **Fat:** 14g **Fiber:** 8g **Sodium:** 450mg

Ingredients:

For the Lemon-Herb Salmon:

4 salmon fillets

2 tablespoons olive oil

2 tablespoons fresh lemon juice

2 cloves garlic, minced

1 teaspoon dried thyme

1 teaspoon dried oregano

A pinch of salt and pepper

For the Caponata & Farro:

1 cup farro, cooked according to package instructions

1 eggplant, diced

1 zucchini, diced

1 bell pepper, diced

1 onion, diced

2 cloves garlic, minced

1 can (14 oz) diced tomatoes

2 tablespoons balsamic vinegar

1 tablespoon honey

1 teaspoon dried basil

A pinch of salt and pepper

Fresh basil leaves for garnish

Method of Preparation:

1. Preheat the oven to 400°F (200°C).

2. In a small bowl, whisk together olive oil, fresh lemon juice, minced garlic, dried thyme, dried oregano, salt, and pepper.

3. Place the salmon fillets on a baking sheet lined with parchment paper. Brush the lemon-herb mixture over the salmon.

4. Bake the salmon in the preheated oven for 12-15 minutes, or until cooked through and flakes easily with a fork.

5. While the salmon is baking, prepare the caponata. Heat olive oil in a large pan over medium heat.

6. Add diced eggplant, zucchini, bell pepper, onion, and minced garlic to the pan. Cook for 8-10 minutes, or until vegetables are softened.

7. Stir in diced tomatoes, balsamic vinegar, honey, dried basil, salt, and pepper. Cook for another 5 minutes.

8. Serve the lemon-herb salmon alongside the caponata and cooked farro. Garnish with fresh basil leaves. Enjoy this flavorful and nutritious meal!

Roasted Salmon with Smoky Chickpeas & Greens

Preparation Time: 35 minutes

Serves: 4

Calories: 340mg **Carbs:** 30g **Protein:** 30g **Fat:** 12g
Fiber: 8g **Sodium:** 400mg

Ingredients:

For the Roasted Salmon:

4 salmon fillets

2 tablespoons olive oil

2 tablespoons smoked paprika

1 teaspoon garlic powder

1 teaspoon onion powder

A pinch of salt and pepper

For the Smoky Chickpeas & Greens:

2 cans (15 oz each) chickpeas, drained and rinsed

2 tablespoons olive oil

1 tablespoon smoked paprika

1 teaspoon cumin

1/2 teaspoon chili powder

A pinch of salt and pepper

4 cups mixed greens (such as spinach, kale, and arugula)

Lemon wedges for serving

Method of Preparation:

1. Preheat the oven to 400°F (200°C).
2. In a small bowl, mix together olive oil, smoked paprika, garlic powder, onion powder, salt, and pepper.
3. Place the salmon fillets on a baking sheet lined with parchment paper. Brush the smoky olive oil mixture over the salmon.
4. Roast the salmon in the preheated oven for 12-15 minutes, or until cooked through and flakes easily with a fork.
5. While the salmon is roasting, prepare the smoky chickpeas. In a large bowl, toss chickpeas with olive

oil, smoked paprika, cumin, chili powder, salt, and pepper until well coated.

6. Spread the chickpeas in a single layer on a baking sheet lined with parchment paper. Roast in the oven for 15-20 minutes, or until crispy.

7. Serve the roasted salmon alongside the smoky chickpeas and mixed greens. Squeeze fresh lemon juice over the salmon before serving. Enjoy this delicious and nutritious meal!

Fish Curry with Noodles

Preparation Time: 45 minutes

Serves: 4

Calories: 320mg **Carbs:** 35g **Protein:** 25g **Fat:** 10g
Fiber: 5g **Sodium:** 500mg

Ingredients:

For the Fish Curry:

1 lb. white fish fillets (such as cod or tilapia), cut into chunks

1 tablespoon olive oil

1 onion, diced

2 cloves garlic, minced

1 tablespoon grated ginger

2 tablespoons curry powder

1 can (14 oz) coconut milk

1 cup vegetable broth

1 tablespoon soy sauce (or tamari for gluten-free)

1 tablespoon lime juice

A pinch of salt and pepper

For the Noodles:

8 oz rice noodles (or any noodles of your choice)

Fresh cilantro for garnish

Lime wedges for serving

Method of Preparation:

1. Cook the noodles according to the package instructions. Drain and set aside.

2. In a large pot, heat olive oil over medium heat. Add diced onion and cook until softened, about 5 minutes.

3. Add minced garlic, grated ginger, and curry powder to the pot. Cook for another 2 minutes, stirring constantly.

4. Stir in coconut milk, vegetable broth, and soy sauce. Bring the mixture to a simmer.

5. Add fish chunks to the pot and simmer for 5-7 minutes, or until the fish is cooked through.

6. Stir in lime juice and season with A pinch of salt and pepper.

7. Serve the fish curry over cooked noodles.

8. Garnish with fresh cilantro and serve with lime wedges on the side. Enjoy this aromatic and flavorful fish curry with noodles!

Prawn Stir Fry with Ginger

Preparation Time: 25 minutes

Serves: 4

Calories: 220mg **Carbs:** 10g **Protein:** 25g **Fat:** 10g
Fiber: 2g **Sodium:** 400mg

Ingredients:

1 lb. prawns, peeled and deveined

2 tablespoons olive oil

2 cloves garlic, minced

1 tablespoon fresh ginger, grated

1 bell pepper, sliced

1 cup snow peas, trimmed

1 carrot, julienned

2 tablespoons soy sauce (or tamari for gluten-free)

1 tablespoon rice vinegar

1 tablespoon honey or maple syrup

1 teaspoon sesame oil

Sesame seeds for garnish

Cooked rice or noodles for serving

Method of Preparation:

1. Heat olive oil in a large pan or wok over medium-high heat.

2. Add minced garlic and grated ginger to the pan. Cook for 1 minute until fragrant.

3. Add prawns to the pan and cook for 2-3 minutes, or until they start to turn pink.

4. Add sliced bell pepper, snow peas, and julienned carrot to the pan. Stir-fry for another 3-4 minutes, or until the vegetables are tender-crisp.

5. In a small bowl, whisk together soy sauce, rice vinegar, honey or maple syrup, and sesame oil.

6. Pour the sauce over the prawn stir-fry and toss to coat evenly.

7. Cook for another 1-2 minutes until the sauce thickens slightly.

8. Remove from heat and sprinkle with sesame seeds for garnish.

9. Serve the prawn stir-fry immediately over cooked rice or noodles. Enjoy this delicious and nutritious dish!

Fish Pie

Preparation Time: 60 minutes

Serves: 6

Calories: 380mg **Carbs:** 30g **Protein:** 25g **Fat:** 18g **Fiber:** 4g **Sodium:** 450mg

Ingredients:

For the Fish Filling:

1 lb. white fish fillets (such as cod or haddock), cut into chunks

1 onion, diced

2 cloves garlic, minced

1 carrot, diced

1 cup frozen peas

1 cup vegetable broth

1 tablespoon olive oil

2 tablespoons all-purpose flour (or gluten-free flour)

1 tablespoon fresh parsley, chopped

A pinch of salt and pepper

For the Mashed Potato Topping:

4 large potatoes, peeled and chopped

1/4 cup milk (or dairy-free alternative)

2 tablespoons unsalted butter (or dairy-free margarine)

A pinch of salt and pepper

Method of Preparation:

1. Preheat the oven to 375°F (190°C).
2. Cook the chopped potatoes in boiling water until tender. Drain and mash with milk, butter, salt, and pepper until smooth. Set aside.
3. In a large pan, heat olive oil over medium heat. Add diced onion and cook until softened, about 5 minutes.
4. Add minced garlic and diced carrot to the pan. Cook for another 2 minutes.
5. Sprinkle all-purpose flour over the vegetables and stir to combine.
6. Gradually pour in vegetable broth while stirring constantly to avoid lumps.
7. Add frozen peas and chopped fish fillets to the pan. Cook for 5-7 minutes, or until the fish is cooked through and the sauce thickens.

8. Stir in chopped fresh parsley and season with A pinch of salt and pepper.

9. Transfer the fish filling to a baking dish.

10. Spread the mashed potato topping evenly over the fish filling.

11. Bake in the preheated oven for 25-30 minutes, or until the top is golden and the filling is bubbly.

12. Remove from the oven and let it cool for a few minutes before serving.

13. Serve the fish pie hot and enjoy this comforting and hearty meal!

SOUPS AND STEWS

Smoked Gouda-Broccoli Soup

Preparation Time: 15 minutes

Cooking Time: 25 minutes

Serves:4 servings

Nutritional Facts (per serving):

Calories: 280mg **Carbs:** 20g **Protein:** 15g **Fat:** 16g **Fiber:** 6g **Sodium:** 600mg

Ingredients:

2 cups broccoli florets

1 onion, chopped

2 cloves garlic, minced

2 tablespoons unsalted butter (or olive oil for a dairy-free option)

2 tablespoons all-purpose flour (or gluten-free flour)

2 cups vegetable broth

1 cup milk (or dairy-free alternative)

1 cup shredded smoked Gouda cheese

A pinch of salt and pepper

Smoked paprika for garnish

Croutons for serving (optional)

Method of Preparation:

1. In a large pot, melt unsalted butter over medium heat. Add chopped onion and minced garlic, and cook until softened, about 5 minutes.

2. Stir in all-purpose flour and cook for another 2 minutes, stirring constantly.

3. Gradually pour in vegetable broth while stirring constantly to avoid lumps.

4. Add broccoli florets to the pot and bring the mixture to a simmer. Cook for 10-15 minutes, or until the broccoli is tender.

5. Use an immersion blender to puree the soup until smooth. Alternatively, transfer the soup to a blender and blend until smooth, then return it to the pot.

6. Stir in milk and shredded smoked Gouda cheese until the cheese is melted and the soup is heated through.

7. Season with A pinch of salt and pepper.

8. Ladle the smoked Gouda-broccoli soup into bowls.

9. Garnish with a sprinkle of smoked paprika and serve with croutons if desired.

10. Enjoy this creamy and flavorful soup as a comforting meal!

Instant Pot Lentil Soup

Preparation Time: 30 minutes

Serves: 6

Calories: 240mg **Carbs:** 40g **Protein:** 15g **Fat:** 2g **Fiber:** 15g **Sodium:** 600mg

Ingredients:

1 cup green lentils, rinsed and drained

1 onion, chopped

2 carrots, diced

2 celery stalks, diced

2 cloves garlic, minced

1 can (14 oz) diced tomatoes

4 cups vegetable broth

1 teaspoon ground cumin

1 teaspoon ground coriander

1/2 teaspoon smoked paprika

A pinch of salt and pepper

Fresh parsley for garnish

Method of Preparation:

1. Place all **Ingredients:** (except for salt, pepper, and fresh parsley) into the Instant Pot.
2. Close the lid and set the valve to the sealing position.
3. Cook on high pressure for 10 minutes.
4. Once the cooking time is complete, allow the pressure to release naturally for 5 minutes, then carefully quick-release any remaining pressure.
5. Open the lid and stir the lentil soup. Season with A pinch of salt and pepper.
6. Ladle the soup into bowls and garnish with fresh parsley.
7. Serve hot and enjoy this nutritious and hearty Instant Pot lentil soup!

Caribbean Fish Stew

Preparation Time: 45 minutes

Serves: 4

Calories: 320mg **Carbs:** 20g **Protein:** 25g **Fat:** 15g **Fiber:** 5g **Sodium:** 550mg

Ingredients:

1 lb. white fish fillets (such as tilapia or snapper), cut into chunks

2 tablespoons olive oil

1 onion, chopped

2 cloves garlic, minced

1 bell pepper, chopped

1 cup diced tomatoes

1 cup coconut milk

1 cup vegetable broth

1 tablespoon curry powder

1 teaspoon ground cumin

1 teaspoon paprika

A pinch of salt and pepper

Fresh cilantro for garnish

Cooked rice or quinoa for serving

Method of Preparation:

1. Heat olive oil in a large pot over medium heat. Add chopped onion and minced garlic, and cook until softened, about 5 minutes.
2. Add chopped bell pepper to the pot and cook for another 3 minutes.
3. Stir in diced tomatoes, coconut milk, vegetable broth, curry powder, ground cumin, paprika, salt, and pepper.
4. Bring the mixture to a simmer and cook for 10 minutes, stirring occasionally.
5. Add fish chunks to the pot and cook for another 5-7 minutes, or until the fish is cooked through and flakes easily with a fork.
6. Taste and adjust seasoning if needed.
7. Serve the Caribbean fish stew hot over cooked rice or quinoa.
8. Garnish with fresh cilantro before serving.
9. Enjoy this flavorful and aromatic Caribbean-inspired fish stew!

Potato Leek Soup

Preparation Time: 45 minutes

Serves: 4

Calories: 220mg **Carbs:** 30g **Protein:** 5g **Fat:** 9g **Fiber:** 4g **Sodium:** 500mg

Ingredients:

3 leeks, white and light green parts only, thinly sliced

3 potatoes, peeled and diced

1 onion, chopped

2 cloves garlic, minced

4 cups vegetable broth

1/2 cup heavy cream (or coconut cream for a dairy-free option)

2 tablespoons unsalted butter (or olive oil for a dairy-free option)

A pinch of salt and pepper

Fresh chives for garnish

Method of Preparation:

1. In a large pot, melt unsalted butter over medium heat. Add chopped onion and minced garlic, and cook until softened, about 5 minutes.
2. Add sliced leeks to the pot and cook for another 5 minutes, stirring occasionally.
3. Stir in diced potatoes and vegetable broth. Bring the mixture to a simmer and cook for 15-20 minutes, or until the potatoes are tender.
4. Use an immersion blender to puree the soup until smooth. Alternatively, transfer the soup to a blender and blend until smooth, then return it to the pot.
5. Stir in heavy cream and season with A pinch of salt and pepper.
6. Cook for another 5 minutes, stirring occasionally.
7. Ladle the potato leek soup into bowls.
8. Garnish with fresh chives before serving.
9. Enjoy this creamy and comforting potato leek soup as a delightful meal!

Split Pea Soup with Chorizo

Preparation Time: 1 hour, 45 minutes

Serves: 6

Calories: 320mg **Carbs:** 30g **Protein:** 20g **Fat:** 15g

Fiber: 12g **Sodium:** 800mg

Ingredients:

1 lb. dried split peas, rinsed and drained

1 onion, chopped

2 carrots, diced

2 celery stalks, diced

2 cloves garlic, minced

6 cups chicken or vegetable broth

8 oz chorizo sausage, sliced

2 bay leaves

1 teaspoon dried thyme

A pinch of salt and pepper

Fresh parsley for garnish

Method of Preparation:

1. In a large pot, heat olive oil over medium heat. Add chopped onion, diced carrots, diced celery, and

minced garlic, and cook until softened, about 5 minutes.

2. Add dried split peas, chicken or vegetable broth, bay leaves, dried thyme, salt, and pepper to the pot. Stir to combine.

3. Bring the mixture to a boil, then reduce the heat to low and simmer for 1 hour, stirring occasionally.

4. In a separate pan, cook sliced chorizo sausage until browned and crispy, about 5 minutes.

5. Once the split peas are tender and the soup has thickened, remove the bay leaves from the pot.

6. Use an immersion blender to partially puree the soup, leaving some chunks of split peas for texture. Alternatively, transfer a portion of the soup to a blender and blend until smooth, then return it to the pot.

7. Stir in the cooked chorizo sausage.

8. Taste and adjust seasoning if needed.

9. Serve the split pea soup hot, garnished with fresh parsley.

10. Enjoy this hearty and flavorful split pea soup with chorizo!

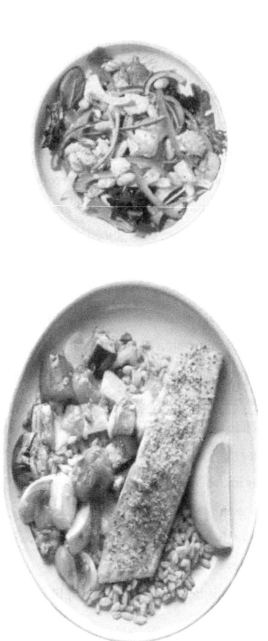

CONCLUSION

In navigating the process of crafting a chemotherapy-friendly cookbook specially for you, it's evident that food can be a powerful ally in the battle against cancer.

Each recipe presented herein embodies a commitment to nourishing the body while considering the unique dietary needs and challenges often associated with cancer treatment.

Embracing ingredients rich in anti-inflammatory properties, low in sodium, and gluten-free, these dishes not only support your overall health but also aid in managing common side effects of chemotherapy, such as inflammation and digestive discomfort.

By emphasizing on nutrient-dense foods such as lean proteins, whole grains, and an abundance of colorful fruits and vegetables, these recipes provide essential vitamins, minerals, and antioxidants vital for promoting healing, boosting immunity, and enhancing overall well-being during treatment and recovery.

Beyond the nutritional benefits, these recipes are designed with practicality in mind, offering straightforward

preparation methods and readily available ingredients. This ensures that even during challenging times, you can easily incorporate nourishing meals into your daily routine without added stress or complication.

Finally, this cookbook serves as a proof to the transformative power of food as medicine during chemotherapy. Always remember to contact a dietician and your doctor for professional advice.

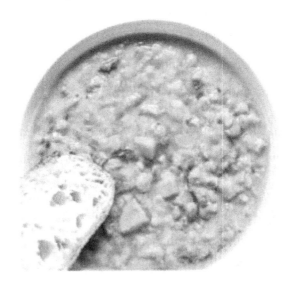

Made in the USA
Las Vegas, NV
18 December 2024

14620743R00066